Apple Cider Vinegar, Coconut Oil and Almond Oil for Beginners

Health and Beauty Secrets Revealed

Disclaimer and Terms of Use:

Effort has been made to ensure that the information in this book is accurate and complete, however, the author and the publisher do not warrant the accuracy of the information, text and graphics contained within the book due to the rapidly changing nature of science, research, known and unknown facts and internet. The Author and the publisher do not hold any responsibility for errors, omissions or contrary interpretation of the subject matter herein. This book is presented solely for motivational and informational purposes only.

Table of Contents

Introduction

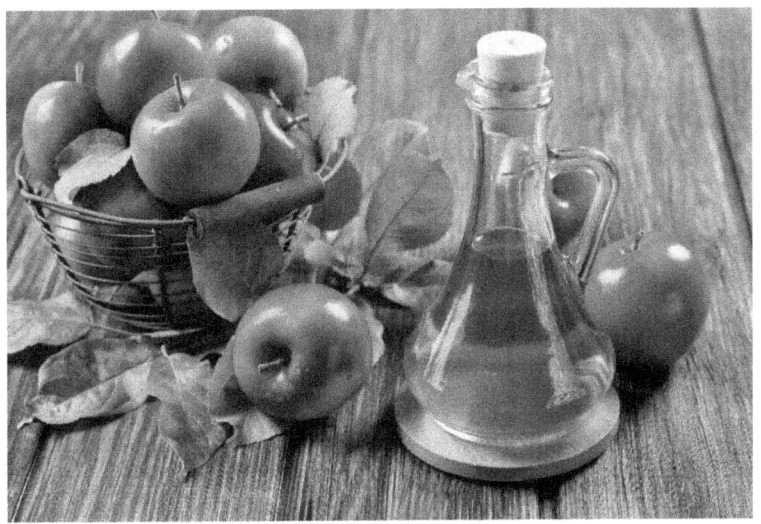

When it comes to keeping your skin, hair and nails healthy and beautiful, you may think that expensive organic beauty products are the only option. While it is true that organic beauty products can work wonders for your body, you don't necessarily have to spend a fortune on them. In fact, you may be able to make them right in your own home! What is the secret? Three powerful ingredients – apple cider vinegar, coconut oil, and almond oil. These ingredients are the foundation of many organic beauty products that you can use to restore the suppleness of your skin, the shine of your hair, and the strength of your nails. These ingredients can also be used in natural remedies to cure common ailments. All three of these ingredients can be purchased at your local grocery or health food store and, combined with a few other simple ingredients, they can be used to make homemade organic beauty products. So, if you are ready to restore your health and boost your beauty, keep reading!

Apple Cider Vinegar, Coconut Oil, and Almond Oil Recipes

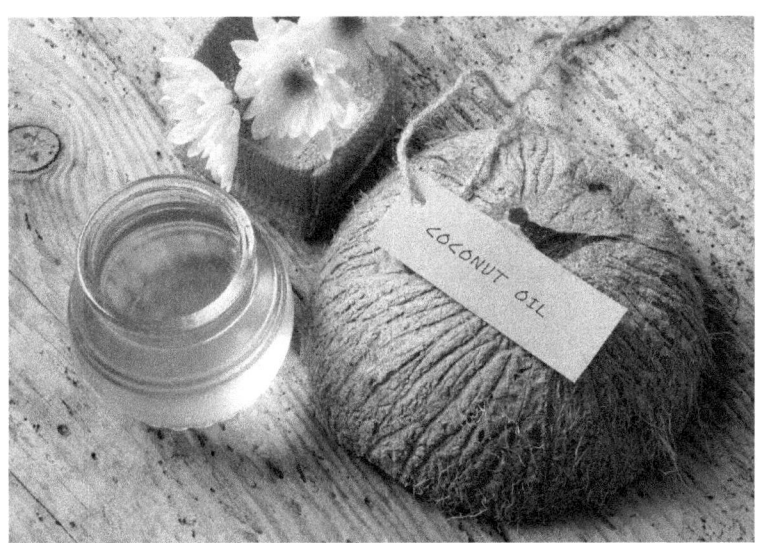

Recipes Included in this Book:

Apple Cider Vinegar Acne Wash

Almond Oil Remedy for Constipation

Itch-Relieving Coconut Oil Paste

Apple Cider Vinegar Liniment for Arthritis

Congestion-Reducing Chest Rub

Dandruff-Reducing Almond Oil Treatment

Blood Pressure-Reducing Vinegar Tonic

Apple Cider Vinegar Burn Treatment

Invigorating Almond Oil Tonic

Soothing Coconut Oil Sunburn Ointment

Immune-Boosting Tonic

Nail Fungus Apple Cider Vinegar Treatment

Bad Breath-Busting Cider Vinegar Rinse

Coconut Oil Eczema Relief Cream

Moisturizing Lavender Salve

Coconut Oil Pull to Whiten Teeth

Spiced Honey Lip Balm

Almond Coconut Milk Shampoo

Rosemary Coconut Oil Lotion Bars

Homemade Coconut Oil Deodorant

Simple Cider Vinegar Hair Rinse

Almond Oil Lotion

Coconut Oil Hand Cream

Coconut and Almond Oil Lye Soap

Rejuvenating Citrus Bath Salts

Coconut Oil Deep Conditioner

Apple Cider Vinegar Shampoo

Minty Whipped Coconut Oil Body Butter

Vanilla Jasmine Lye Soap

Coconut Oil Sugar Scrub

Apple Cider Vinegar Facial Toner

Calming Lavender Rosemary Bath Salts

Holiday Spice Lotion Bar

Lovely Lemon Lip Balm

Floral Whipped Body Butter

Mango Butter Hand Cream

Brown Sugar Coconut Oil Scrub

Natural Remedies

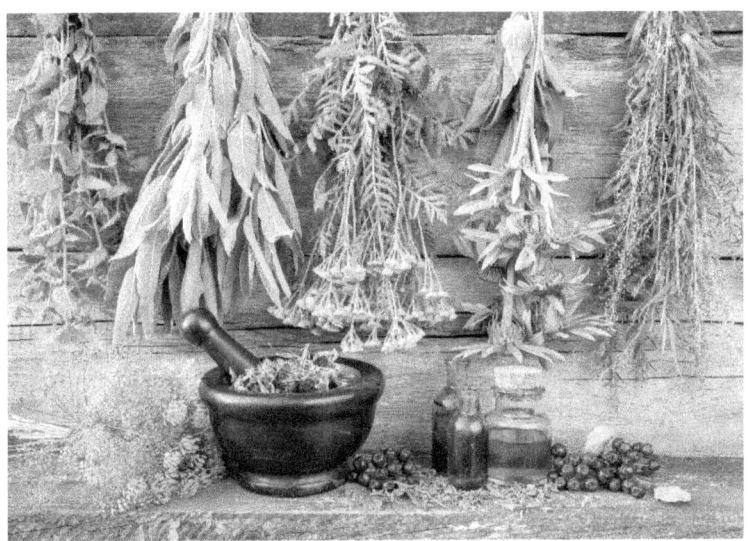

<u>Recipes Included in this Section</u>:

Apple Cider Vinegar Acne Wash

Almond Oil Remedy for Constipation

Itch-Relieving Coconut Oil Paste

Apple Cider Vinegar Liniment for Arthritis

Congestion-Reducing Chest Rub

Dandruff-Reducing Almond Oil Treatment

Blood Pressure-Reducing Vinegar Tonic

Apple Cider Vinegar Burn Treatment

Invigorating Almond Oil Tonic

Soothing Coconut Oil Sunburn Ointment

Immune-Boosting Tonic

Nail Fungus Apple Cider Vinegar Treatment

Bad Breath-Busting Cider Vinegar Rinse

Coconut Oil Eczema Relief Cream

Moisturizing Lavender Salve

Apple Cider Vinegar Acne Wash

Ingredients:

- 8 ounces filtered water

- 2 tablespoons organic apple cider vinegar

- Cotton balls

Instructions:

1. Pour the water into a bowl and add the apple cider vinegar.

2. Stir well then pour the mixture into a glass jar to store at room temperature.

3. Soak a cotton ball in the mixture and squeeze out the extra liquid.

4. Apply the cotton ball to skin affected by acne to reduce inflammation and redness.

5. Use the mixture several times per day to reduce infection and heal acne.

Almond Oil Remedy for Constipation

Ingredients:

- 6 ounces plain Greek yogurt

- 1 tablespoon organic almond oil

- 1 tablespoon raw honey

Instructions:

1. Place the yogurt in a small bowl then add the almond oil.

2. Stir in the honey until the mixture is smooth and well combined.

3. Enjoy the yogurt for breakfast or as a snack to soothe digestive upset and reduce constipation.

Itch-Relieving Coconut Oil Paste

Ingredients:

- 1 tablespoon organic coconut oil

- 1 tablespoon baking soda

Instructions:

1. Combine the coconut oil and baking soda in a small bowl.

2. Stir the mixture into a thick paste using a fork.

3. Apply a small amount of the paste to bug bites or other irritated areas to relieve itching and to reduce inflammation.

Apple Cider Vinegar Liniment for Arthritis

Ingredients:

- 2 large egg whites, beaten

- ½ cup organic apple cider vinegar

- ¼ cup organic olive oil

Instructions:

1. Beat the egg whites in a small bowl until frothy.

2. Add the apple cider vinegar and olive oil, whisking until smooth.

3. Massage the mixture into sore joints for 30 to 60 seconds once a day.

Congestion-Reducing Chest Rub

Ingredients:

- ¼ cup organic coconut oil
- 2 tablespoons beeswax granules
- 1 ½ tablespoons sweet almond oil
- ½ teaspoon eucalyptus essential oil
- ½ teaspoon lavender essential oil

Instructions:

1. Combine the coconut oil and beeswax in a double boiler until melted.
2. Remove from heat and cool to room temperature.
3. Combine the sweet almond oil and essential oils in a small glass jar.
4. Pour in the melted oil and beeswax then stir well.

5. Place the jar in the refrigerator until the mixture solidifies.

6. Rub a small amount of the mixture into the skin on your chest as needed to relieve chest congestion.

Dandruff-Reducing Almond Oil Treatment

Ingredients:

- Organic almond oil, as needed

Instructions:

1. Apple a small amount of almond oil to your scalp.

2. Massage the almond oil into your hair and scalp with your fingers.

3. Let the mixture rest for 30 minutes then wash with warm water and towel dry.

4. Repeat the treatment three times a week until the dandruff is gone.

Blood Pressure-Reducing Vinegar Tonic

Ingredients:

- 8 ounces filtered water

- 1 tablespoon organic apple cider vinegar

- 1 tablespoon raw honey

Instructions:

1. Pour the water into a bowl and add the apple cider vinegar and honey.

2. Stir well then pour the mixture into a glass.

3. Drink the tonic twice per day to help lower blood pressure naturally.

4. To increase the benefits of this tonic, combine with a low-sodium diet and increased fiber intake.

Apple Cider Vinegar Burn Treatment

Ingredients:

- Cold water, as needed

- 2 tablespoons organic apple cider vinegar

- Cotton balls

Instructions:

1. Run cold water over the burned area for at least 5 minutes.

2. Pour the apple cider vinegar into a small bowl.

3. Dip a cotton ball in the vinegar then squeeze out the excess liquid.

4. Apply the cotton ball to the burned area to disinfect, reduce pain, and start healing.

Invigorating Almond Oil Tonic

Ingredients:

- 1 ½ cups unsweetened almond milk

- 2 tablespoons unsweetened cocoa powder

- 1 tablespoon organic coconut oil

- 1 tablespoon chia seeds

- 1 tablespoons ground flaxseed

- 1 tablespoon raw honey

- 1 teaspoon organic almond oil

- ½ teaspoon ground cinnamon

- ¼ teaspoon ground turmeric

- Pinch sea salt

Instructions:

1. Combine all of the ingredients in a high-speed

   blender.

2. Pulse the mixture several times then blend on high

    speed until smooth.

3. Pour the mixture into a glass filled with ice to

    serve.

4. Alternatively, warm the mixture in a saucepan on

    the stove and serve in a mug.

Soothing Coconut Oil Sunburn Ointment

Ingredients:

- ¼ cup organic coconut oil

- 1 tablespoon aloe vera

- 1 tablespoon raw honey

Instructions:

1. Place the coconut oil in a small glass jar.

2. Put the jar in a bowl or saucepan of hot water and let the coconut oil melt.

3. Stir the aloe vera and honey into the jar then remove from the bowl.

4. Allow the mixture to sit at room temperature for a few minutes until it starts to solidify.

5. Rub a small amount of the ointment into sunburned skin as needed.

Immune-Boosting Tonic

Ingredients:

- 2 tablespoons minced garlic

- 2 tablespoons fresh grated ginger

- 2 tablespoons fresh grated horseradish

- 2 tablespoons minced jalapeno

- 2 tablespoons minced white onion

- 1 tablespoon organic almond oil

- Organic apple cider vinegar, as needed

Instructions:

1. Combine all of the ingredients in large glass jar,

   filling it about ¾ full.

2. Pour in enough apple cider vinegar to fill the jar.

3. Cover the jar with the lid and let it set for 2 weeks

   in a cool, dark area at room temperature.

4. Strain the liquid from the jar into a separate glass

    jar.

5. To use, stir 1 to 2 tablespoons of the liquid into 8

    ounces of water and drink twice daily.

Nail Fungus Apple Cider Vinegar Treatment

Ingredients:

- Warm water, as needed
- 1 cup organic apple cider vinegar
- 5 tablespoons baking soda

Instructions:

1. Fill a plastic tub with warm water then stir in the apple cider vinegar.
2. Soak your feet in the water for about 15 minutes then towel dry.
3. Empty the tub and refill it with warm water.
4. Stir in the baking soda then soak your feet for 15 minutes then towel dry.

5. Perform this remedy twice per day until the fungus goes away.

6. The vinegar will help to kill it while the baking soda prevents it from growing back.

Bad Breath-Busting Cider Vinegar Rinse

Ingredients:

- 8 ounces filtered water

- 1 tablespoon organic apple cider vinegar

Instructions:

1. Combine the water and cider vinegar in a glass.

2. Drink the liquid after consuming a meal to reduce bad breath.

Coconut Oil Eczema Relief Cream

Ingredients:

- 5 tablespoons organic coconut oil

- ½ tablespoon vitamin E oil

- 2 teaspoons rosemary oil

Instructions:

1. Spoon the coconut oil into a small glass jar.

2. Place the jar in a bowl of hot water until the coconut oil melts.

3. Stir in the vitamin E oil and rosemary oil until smooth.

4. Spread the mixture over the affected area and let it set for 5 minutes.

5. Rinse with warm water and pat dry.

Moisturizing Lavender Salve

Ingredients:

- 3 tablespoons organic coconut oil

- 1 teaspoon vitamin E oil

- 8 drops lavender essential oil

- 4 drops tea tree essential oil

Instructions:

1. Place the coconut oil in a small bowl and warm it in the microwave until melted.

2. Add the essential oils and vitamin E oil then stir until well combined.

3. Pour the mixture into a small glass jar and let sit at room temperature until solidified.

4. Apply the salve directly to your skin as needed to soothe and moisturize.

Organic Homemade Beauty Products

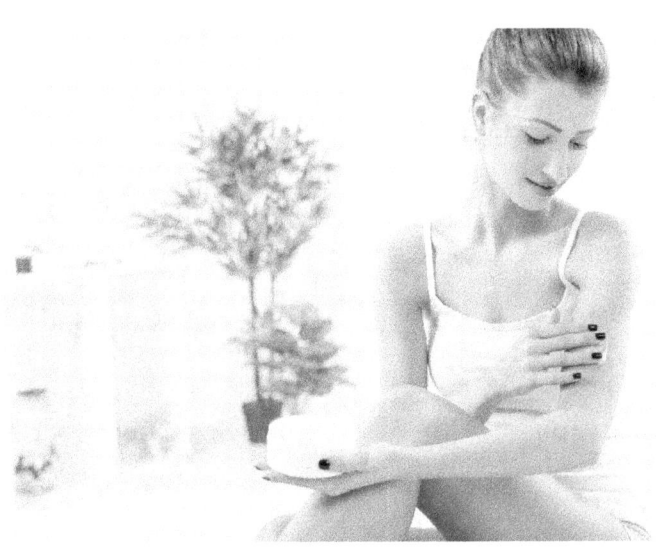

Recipes Included in this Section:

Coconut Oil Pull to Whiten Teeth

Spiced Honey Lip Balm

Almond Coconut Milk Shampoo

Rosemary Coconut Oil Lotion Bars

Homemade Coconut Oil Deodorant

Simple Cider Vinegar Hair Rinse

Almond Oil Lotion

Coconut Oil Hand Cream

Coconut and Almond Oil Lye Soap

Rejuvenating Citrus Bath Salts

Coconut Oil Deep Conditioner

Apple Cider Vinegar Shampoo

Minty Whipped Coconut Oil Body Butter

Vanilla Jasmine Lye Soap

Coconut Oil Sugar Scrub

Apple Cider Vinegar Facial Toner

Calming Lavender Rosemary Bath Salts

Holiday Spice Lotion Bars

Lovely Lemon Lip Balm

Floral Whipped Body Butter

Mango Butter Hand Cream

Brown Sugar Coconut Oil Scrub

Coconut Oil Pull to Whiten Teeth

Ingredients:

- 2 tablespoons organic coconut oil

Instructions:

1. Melt the coconut oil in a microwave-safe bowl at 10-second intervals until melted.

2. Spoon the melted oil into your mouth after making sure it isn't too hot.

3. Swish the oil in your mouth and between your teeth for about 10 to 20 minutes.

4. Avoid swallowing any of the oil and swish gently.

5. Spit the oil out then immediately rinse your mouth with warm salt water.

6. Brush your teeth as you normally would – this is best done first thing in the morning.

Spiced Honey Lip Balm

Ingredients:

- 2 tablespoons organic coconut oil

- 2 tablespoons beeswax granules

- 1 tablespoon shea butter

- 1 teaspoon raw honey

- 3 teaspoons sweet almond oil

- 6 drops cinnamon essential oil

- 4 drops clove essential oil

- 2 drops ginger essential oil

Instructions:

1. Combine the coconut oil, beeswax, shea butter, and honey in a double boiler.

2. Heat the mixture until melted then remove from heat.

3. Stir in the sweet almond oil and essential oils until well combined.

4. Pour the mixture into empty lip balm tubes and set them upright.

5. Allow the lip balm to set then put the caps on the tubes and use the balm as needed.

Almond Coconut Milk Shampoo

Ingredients:

- ¾ cups liquid castile soap, unscented

- ½ cup canned coconut milk

- 1 teaspoon sweet almond oil

- 12 drops tea tree essential oil

- 6 to 8 drops lavender essential oil

Instructions:

1. Pour all of the ingredients into a mixing bowl and stir well.

2. Transfer the mixture to an empty shampoo bottle.

3. Shake the bottle then apply a small amount of shampoo to damp hair in the shower.

4. Work the shampoo into a lather then rinse and condition as desired.

Rosemary Coconut Oil Lotion Bars

Ingredients:

- 1 cup organic coconut oil
- 1 cup organic shea butter
- 1 cup beeswax granules
- 1 teaspoon vitamin E oil
- 4 to 6 drops rosemary essential oil

Instructions:

1. Combine the coconut oil, shea butter and beeswax in a double boiler over low heat.
2. Heat until the ingredients are melted then remove from heat and stir smooth.
3. Stir in the vitamin E oil and rosemary essential oil until well combined.

4. Pour the mixture into silicone baking molds or mini muffin pans lined with paper liners.

5. Allow the lotion bars to cool until firm then remove from the molds.

Homemade Coconut Oil Deodorant

Ingredients:

- 3 tablespoons organic coconut oil

- 2 tablespoons organic sea butter

- 3 tablespoons baking soda

- 2 tablespoons arrowroot powder

- 3 drops lavender essential oil

- 2 drops tea tree essential oil

Instructions:

1. Melt the coconut oil and shea butter in a double boiler over medium-low heat.

2. Once the ingredients are melted, stir smooth then remove from heat.

3. Stir in the baking soda and arrowroot powder.

4. Add the essential oils then stir well and pour into a small glass jar.

5. Allow the deodorant to solidify at room temperature.

6. Apply the deodorant as needed once a day.

Simple Cider Vinegar Hair Rinse

Ingredients:

- ½ cup organic apple cider vinegar

- ½ cup warm filtered water

Instructions:

1. Pour both of the ingredients into a mixing bowl and stir well.

2. Transfer the mixture to an empty plastic spray bottle.

3. Wash your hair as you normally would then spray with the hair rinse.

4. Massage the mixture into your scalp and let it set for 3 minutes.

5. Rinse with warm water then towel dry.

Almond Oil Lotion

Ingredients:

- ½ cup organic sweet almond oil

- ¼ cup organic coconut oil

- 3 tablespoons organic shea butter

- ¼ cup beeswax granules

- ½ teaspoon organic almond extract

Instructions:

1. Combine the almond oil, coconut oil and cocoa butter in a double boiler over low heat.

2. Heat until the ingredients are melted then remove from heat and stir smooth.

3. Stir in the beeswax and almond extract until well combined.

4. Spoon the mixture into a small glass jar and allow it

    to solidify at room temperature.

5. Use the lotion daily to nourish and heal dry skin.

Coconut Oil Hand Cream

Ingredients:

- ½ cup organic coconut oil

- ¼ cup organic cocoa butter

- ¼ cup organic shea butter

- 1 ½ tablespoons sweet almond oil

- 1 teaspoon vitamin E oil

- 4 to 6 drops essential oil (your choice)

Instructions:

1. Combine the coconut oil, cocoa butter, and shea butter in a double boiler over low heat.

2. Heat until the ingredients are melted then remove from heat and stir smooth.

3. Stir in the sweet almond oil, vitamin E oil, and essential oil until well combined.

4. Pour the mixture into silicone baking molds or mini muffin pans lined with paper liners.

5. Allow the lotion bars to cool until firm then remove from the molds.

Coconut and Almond Oil Lye Soap

Ingredients:

- ¾ cups filtered water

- ¼ cup liquid lye

- 1 cup organic coconut oil

- 2/3 cups sweet almond oil

- 1/3 cup organic olive oil

- Essential oils, if desired

Instructions:

1. Pour the water into a large glass jar then carefully stir in the lye.

2. Stir until the mixture starts to clear then set it aside.

3. In a separate jar, combine the coconut oil, almond oil and olive oil.

4. Place the jar in a saucepan of simmering water until melted then pour into a bowl.

5. Whisk in the lye mixture very slowly and stir for about 5 minutes.

6. Blend the mixture using an immersion blender until thick then blend in the essential oils.

7. Pour the soap mixture into soap molds then cover with plastic.

8. Wrap the molds in a clean towel and let rest at room temperature for 24 hours.

9. Remove the soap from the molds and cut into bars.

10. Let the bars cure for about 4 weeks, turning them once per week.

Rejuvenating Citrus Bath Salts

Ingredients:

- 2 cups coarse sea salts

- 1 tablespoon sweet almond oil

- 15 drops sweet orange essential oil

- 10 drops lemon essential oil

- 5 drops grapefruit essential oil

Instructions:

1. Place the salt in a medium-sized bowl.

2. Add the sweet almond oil and the essential oils then stir well to combine.

3. Store the salts in a glass jar or airtight container.

4. Add ¼ to ½ cup of the salts to running bath water then stir gently by hand.

5. Soak in the bath for at least 30 minutes then towel dry.

Coconut Oil Deep Conditioner

Ingredients:

- Organic coconut oil, as needed

Instructions:

1. Apply a tablespoon of coconut oil to dry hair.

2. Carefully comb the oil through your hair then gather it into a loose bun.

3. Put on a shower cap then sleep with the oil in your hair.

4. In the morning, wash your hair as you normally would with shampoo.

Apple Cider Vinegar Shampoo

Ingredients:

- 1 cup unscented liquid castile soap

- ¼ cup warm filtered water

- 2 tablespoons organic apple cider vinegar

- 1 teaspoon vitamin E oil

- 10 to 14 drops tea tree essential oil

Instructions:

1. Pour all of the ingredients into a mixing bowl and stir well.

2. Transfer the mixture to an empty shampoo bottle.

3. Shake the bottle then apply a small amount of shampoo to damp hair in the shower.

4. Work the shampoo into a lather then rinse and condition as desired.

Minty Whipped Coconut Oil Body Butter

Ingredients:

- 1 cup organic coconut oil

- ½ cup cocoa butter

- ½ cup sweet almond oil

- 16 drops peppermint essential oil

Instructions:

1. Combine the coconut oil and cocoa butter in a double boiler.

2. Heat until the ingredients are melted then stir smooth.

3. Remove from heat and whisk in the almond oil and peppermint essential oil.

4. Pour the mixture into a bowl then chill for 1 hour until it starts to solidify.

5. Beat the mixture with a hand mixer on high speed until fluffy – about 8 to 10 minutes.

6. Place the bowl back in the fridge for 10 minutes then store in a glass jar.

Vanilla Jasmine Lye Soap

Ingredients:

- ¾ cups filtered water

- ¼ cup liquid lye

- 1 cup organic coconut oil

- 2/3 cups sweet almond oil

- 1/3 cup organic olive oil

- ½ teaspoon vanilla essential oil

- ¼ teaspoon jasmine essential oil

Instructions:

1. Pour the water into a large glass jar then carefully stir in the lye.

2. Stir until the mixture starts to clear then set it aside.

3. In a separate jar, combine the coconut oil, almond oil and olive oil.

4. Place the jar in a saucepan of simmering water until melted then pour into a bowl.

5. Whisk in the lye mixture very slowly and stir for about 5 minutes.

6. Blend the mixture using an immersion blender until thick then blend in the essential oils.

7. Pour the soap mixture into soap molds then cover with plastic.

8. Wrap the molds in a clean towel and let rest at room temperature for 24 hours.

9. Remove the soap from the molds and cut into bars.

10. Let the bars cure for about 4 weeks, turning them once per week.

Coconut Oil Sugar Scrub

Ingredients:

- ½ cup organic coconut oil

- ¼ cup organic cane sugar

- 1 tablespoon fresh orange zest

- 20 drops orange essential oil

- 15 drops lemon essential oil

Instructions:

1. Combine the ingredients in a small glass jar.

2. Stir until thoroughly combined and store at room temperature with the lid on.

3. To use, apply a small amount of the scrub to damp skin.

4. Rub the scrub into your skin for 1 minute then rinse with cool water and pat dry.

Apple Cider Vinegar Facial Toner

Ingredients:

- ¼ cup warm filtered water

- 2 tablespoons organic apple cider vinegar

Instructions:

1. Whisk together the ingredients in a small bowl.

2. Pour into a small glass jar and store at room temperature.

3. To apply the toner, soak a cotton ball in the liquid then squeeze to remove moisture.

4. Dab the toner onto your skin after washing.

Calming Lavender Rosemary Bath Salts

Ingredients:

- 2 cups coarse Himalayan pink salt

- 1 tablespoon sweet almond oil

- 15 drops lavender essential oil

- 10 drops rosemary essential oil

Instructions:

1. Place the salt in a medium-sized bowl.

2. Add the sweet almond oil and the essential oils then stir well to combine.

3. Store the salts in a glass jar or airtight container.

4. Add ¼ to ½ cup of the salts to running bath water then stir gently by hand.

5. Soak in the bath for at least 30 minutes then towel dry.

Holiday Spice Lotion Bars

Ingredients:

- 1 cup organic coconut oil

- 1 cup organic shea butter

- 1 cup beeswax granules

- 1 teaspoon vitamin E oil

- 6 drops pine essential oil

- 4 drops cedarwood essential oil

- 2 drops clove essential oil

Instructions:

1. Combine the coconut oil, shea butter and beeswax in a double boiler over low heat.

2. Heat until the ingredients are melted then remove from heat and stir smooth.

3. Stir in the vitamin E oil and essential oils until well combined.

4. Pour the mixture into silicone baking molds or mini muffin pans lined with paper liners.

5. Allow the lotion bars to cool until firm then remove from the molds.

Lovely Lemon Lip Balm

Ingredients:

- 2 tablespoons organic coconut oil

- 2 tablespoons beeswax granules

- 1 tablespoon cocoa butter

- 1 teaspoon raw honey

- 3 teaspoons sweet almond oil

- 1 teaspoon fresh lemon zest

- 12 drops lemon essential oil

Instructions:

1. Combine the coconut oil, beeswax, cocoa butter, and honey in a double boiler.

2. Heat the mixture until melted then remove from heat.

3. Stir in the sweet almond oil, lemon zest, and lemon essential oil until well combined.

4. Pour the mixture into empty lip balm tubes and set them upright.

5. Allow the lip balm to set then put the caps on the tubes and use the balm as needed.

Floral Whipped Body Butter

Ingredients:

- 1 cup organic coconut oil

- ½ cup cocoa butter

- ½ cup sweet almond oil

- 8 drops jasmine essential oil

- 6 drops rose essential oil

- 2 drops lavender essential oil

Instructions:

1. Combine the coconut oil and cocoa butter in a double boiler.

2. Heat until the ingredients are melted then stir smooth.

3. Remove from heat and whisk in the almond oil and essential oils.

4. Pour the mixture into a bowl then chill for 1 hour until it starts to solidify.

5. Beat the mixture with a hand mixer on high speed until fluffy – about 8 to 10 minutes.

6. Place the bowl back in the fridge for 10 minutes then store in a glass jar.

Mango Butter Hand Cream

Ingredients:

- ½ cup organic coconut oil
- ½ cup organic mango butter
- 2 tablespoons sweet almond oil
- 1 teaspoon vitamin E oil
- 4 to 6 drops essential oil (your choice)

Instructions:

1. Combine the coconut oil and mango butter in a double boiler over low heat.
2. Heat until the ingredients are melted then remove from heat and stir smooth.
3. Stir in the sweet almond oil, vitamin E oil, and essential oil until well combined.

4. Pour the mixture into silicone baking molds or mini muffin pans lined with paper liners.

5. Allow the lotion bars to cool until firm then remove from the molds.

Brown Sugar Coconut Oil Scrub

Ingredients:

- ½ cup organic coconut oil

- ¼ cup organic brown sugar

- 1 tablespoon fresh lemon zest

- 30 to 50 drops essential oil (your choice)

Instructions:

1. Combine the ingredients in a small glass jar.

2. Stir until thoroughly combined and store at room temperature with the lid on.

3. To use, apply a small amount of the scrub to damp skin.

4. Rub the scrub into your skin for 1 minute then rinse with cool water and pat dry.

Conclusion

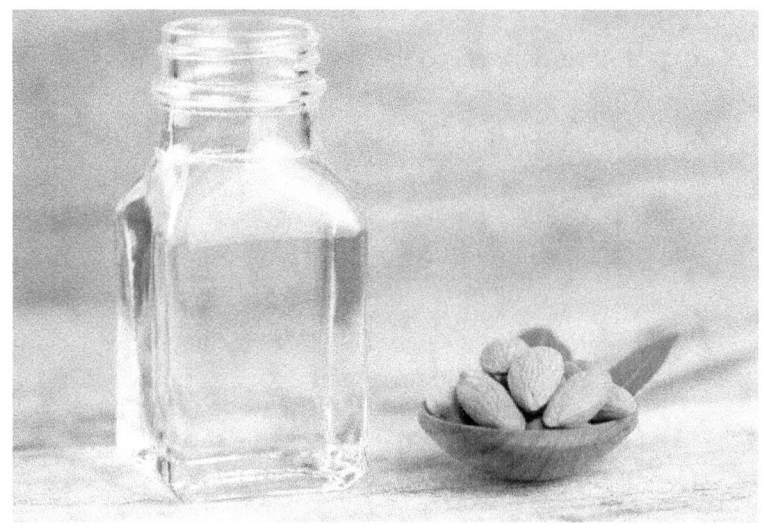

You may not realize it, but the secret to glowing skin, healthy hair, and good health may be sitting in your cupboard right now. Coconut oil, almond oil, and apple cider vinegar are three of the most powerful natural ingredients to use in making your own homemade beauty products and natural remedies. Each of these ingredients has its own unique set of beneficial properties, as you

have seen in reviewing the recipes in this book. If you are

ready to try your hand at homemade organic beauty

products and natural remedies for common ailments,

simply pick a recipe from this book and give it a try!